60 Days to the Real Me...How juice

fasting gave me back my health

By Marc Clarke

For my wonderful family that makes me feel like the most blessed person in the universe. I want to live a healthy and joy filled life with you and inspire you to do the same. Thank you for your amazing support.

I would also like to dedicate this book to the memory of KSwift who inspired with her amazing weight loss and transformation, talent and positive spirit.

Contents

Info & Links

Books:

How to Break a Juice Fast by Carla Douglin with Awanda Baker

101 Juice Fast Recipes by Carla Douglin

Video and Websites:

www.rawrawlife.com

www.marcs60dayfast.com

(a video of the start of the fast with me, Troy, and Carla)

http://youtu.be/LEDoMh3BbLw

(a video of the half-way point with me, Troy, and Carla)

http://youtu.be/kT-WMYUL41E

60 Days to the Real Me...How juice fasting gave me back my health

Before I share my story it's important to let you know that I am not a nutritionist or a doctor. I am just a guy who needed to make a drastic change in my life. The 60 day juice fast was my method of hitting the proverbial restart button to reverse decades of yo-yo diets, overeating and lack of control when it came to food. Please consult with your physician before beginning any weight loss regiment.

THE WAKE UP CALL

What makes you decide to put a life changing decision into action? You've talked about it, whatever "it" is, many times before but you never fully put a plan into action and in the end, you failed. So what has to happen to make you stop talking and start doing? I needed to lose weight. I made the decision to lose 100 pounds long before the day my doctor told me I was pre-diabetic. But hearing her diagnosis gave me the fortitude to finally do it, to say "Hell no, I am not going out like that!" My mother has adult onset type two diabetes and I had too much knowledge of what diabetes can do to you. The condition has led to her having a portion of her foot removed, open heart surgery because of the combined effects of high blood pressure and diabetes and thousands of dollars of eye surgery because of this volatile disease. But the history of diabetes runs even deeper in my family. My Grandmother lost both of her legs to diabetes so hearing those words on that day, brought to mind a mental image of me suffering this same fate and even death. At that moment I knew my life would not be the same.

Before I share my story it's important to let you know that I am not a nutritionist, doctor not a dietician. I am just a guy who needed to make a drastic change in my life. The 60 day juice fast was my method of hitting the proverbial restart button to reverse decades of yo yo diets, overeating and lack of control when it came to food. Please consult with your physician before beginning any weight loss regiment.

The doctor's words that day triggered a long standing fear that was planted decades before on the day my Mother told me that she had diabetes. I was ten years old and the news made me an emotional wreck. She told me during a thunderstorm and this news seemed to add to the drama of the moment. My young mind flashed on my grandmother who was forced to use a wheelchair after diabetes robbed her of her legs. Was my Mother going to suffer the same fate? My fears would creep up again later in high school health class. The lesson that day was on diabetes and genetic predisposition. The instructor said that if one of your parents had it, you were probably going to get it also. After the class I asked her about type two diabetes and how I heard that it could be controlled by exercise, managing your weight and diet. Though I persisted, she told me that if my Mother had diabetes it was pretty certain that I would have it also. So now, all these years later, my high school teacher's words were coming to pass. I was staring down the barrel of this crippling, silent killer that slowly saps your health cutting your life short and permanently affecting the quality of your life. I was facing the possibility of getting diabetes. No! Not on my watch.

The real question was how did I get here? I knew that increased weight raised your chances of becoming diabetic so why had I allowed myself to gain so much weight over the years and why was I tipping the scale at more than three hundred thirty pounds?

THE BEGININNG OF THE FOOD ADDICTION

I began using food as a reward and to cope with disappointment as a child. My mother did it, so I did it. I was raised by a single mom who was going through hell at work. She was under an extreme amount of stress and used food to cope. What she didn't know, and we know now, is that the stress levels probably caused her to hold on to fat around her midsection and this stress contributed to her high blood pressure and type two diabetes. We ate out quite a bit as a family. We ate to celebrate good times like a job promotion or good grades and we ate to comfort bad times like a job demotion and bad news like a death in the family. We ate to get out of the house to maybe get a desert and we ate when we were in the house watching television or listening to music. Food was our vice. My Mother didn't really drink or smoke but we got our eat on! What we didn't know is that when you eat at restaurants you are putting yourself in the hands of an industry that does not care about your health. Their first priority is to make money and provide food that tastes good and keeps you coming back, as cheap as they can. You have no idea how they prepare their food, how much salt and oil and fat they use, or how long it's been sitting in the kitchen. You trust your life to a stranger every time you eat out.

THE START OF DIETING

My first weight related issue happened when I was about eight years old and it was time to get a suit. I blogged about it......

(MY HUSKEY ANGEL BLOG)

I guess the first time I realized that I was chubby was in grade school, just a kid. One memory that I'll never forget happened when I was about ten years old. I had outgrown my only suit and needed a new one. But when Mom and I went to the store to buy a new suit but we couldn't find one that fit me. We kept striking out, store after store until we stopped at a shop called "The Hub." That's where we met a young lady I'll call my Lil' fat boy angel. My angel introduced a word into our family's vocabulary that changed my world. My mother described the situation and how we were having problems finding a youth size for me. My angel then said the magical words "Oh, you need a husky." My mother and I looked at each other and said at the same time "husky?" She said the husky size was big enough for a man, but made for a kid. We went to the husky section and sure enough these suits were the perfect size for me. The Hub not only had husky suits, it also had tough skin jeans in all colors! Sometimes at night, I say a prayer for my lil' fat boy angel.

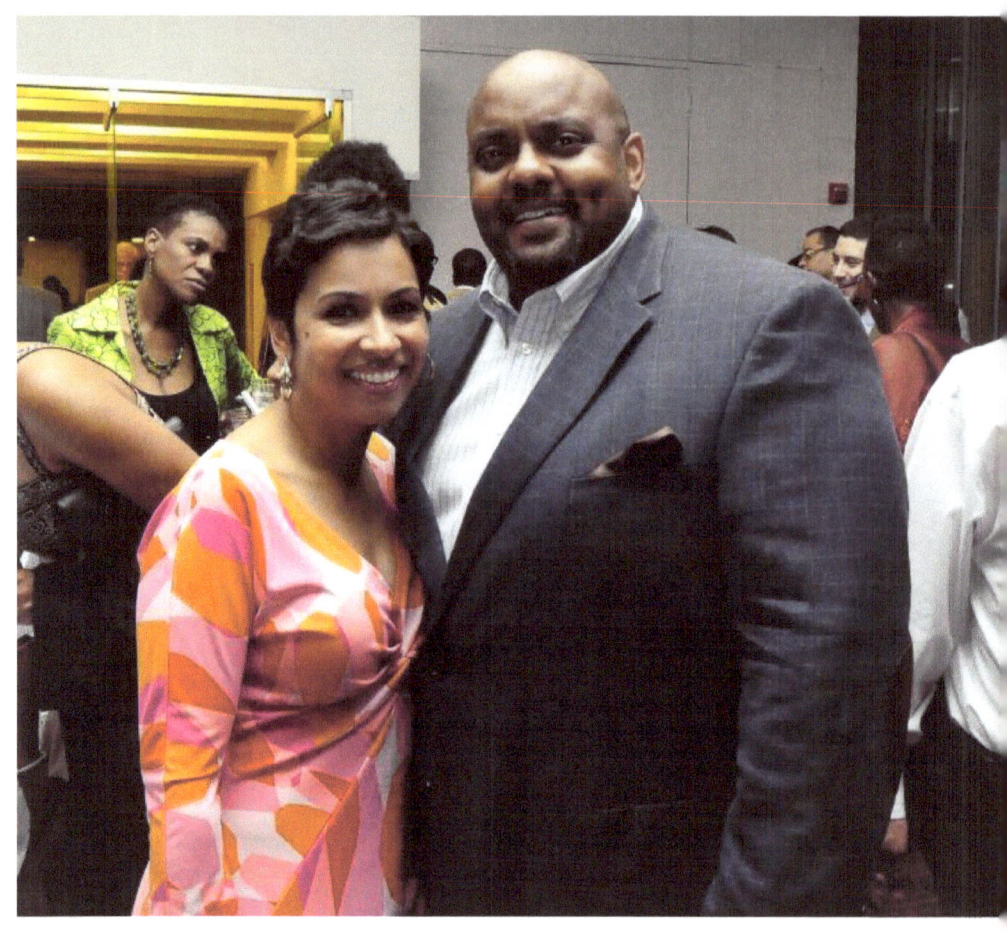

Husky...Again

In seventh grade is when I started my first diet program or workout...I blogged about it:

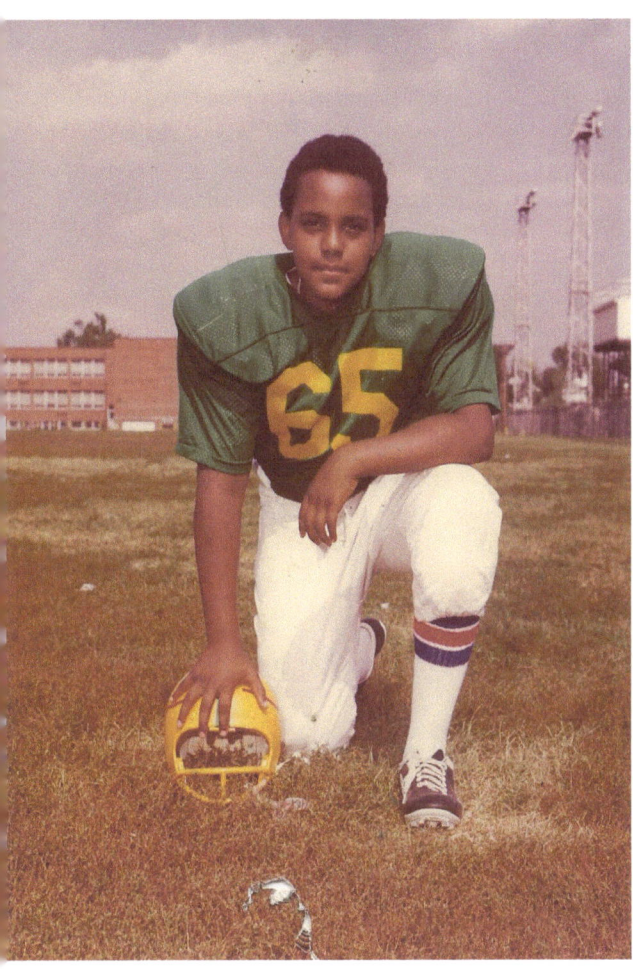

Striper

When I played pee wee football nobody wanted to be a striper. A striper is what they called you when you had a red stripe around your helmet and it meant that you weighed more than 140 pounds and you could not advance the football in any way. If you came in contact with the ball it was instantly ruled dead. The league did not want your 140 pounds pulverizing or maiming the smaller kids. Your dreams of being an offensive superstar went out the window as soon as the scale read 140 pounds or more. As you can see if you look closely at the picture I was a "striper." I hated it. My favorite players were running backs; Franco Harris, O.J. Simpson and Earl Campbell. I wanted to be like them. I wanted to thrill the fans with my break-away speed and shifty moves and if need be, plow over the defenders with my power. With that stripe on my helmet all I could do was plow into the other linemen. So, I approached my coach and asked if I got under 135 pounds the next year could I play running back and he said yes. So this began my first diet and weight loss program. I became the Rocky of my neighborhood. Each evening around 7pm I would put on my sweats and get my run, do push-ups, sit-ups and all the other ups I could do. I trained all winter and when the next season rolled around, my hard work had paid off. I weighed in at a fit 135 and became the starting fullback. It was the first time had set a physical goal and achieved it and it felt great. It also started my interest in weightlifting and fitness. I found that I liked the feeling of building my strength. It gave me confidence. I still use this lesson I learned decades ago to motivate me to achieve new goals.

Did we have a great season once I was able to run the ball? No, I was mediocre and we never won a game... but at least I wasn't a striper. Remember, you don't have to be a striper; you have the power within to be that person you've always wanted to be.

I shared my striper story with musician Branford Marsalis when he was in the studio with us years ago and he gave me this picture which I will always treasure.

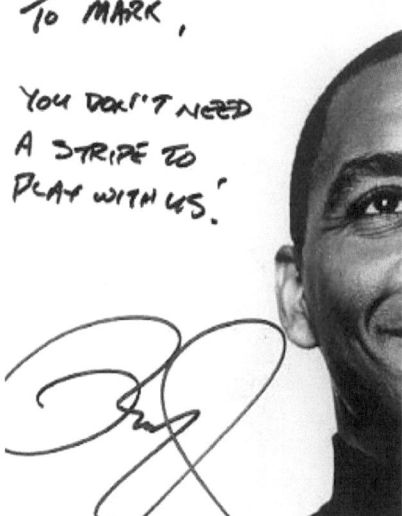

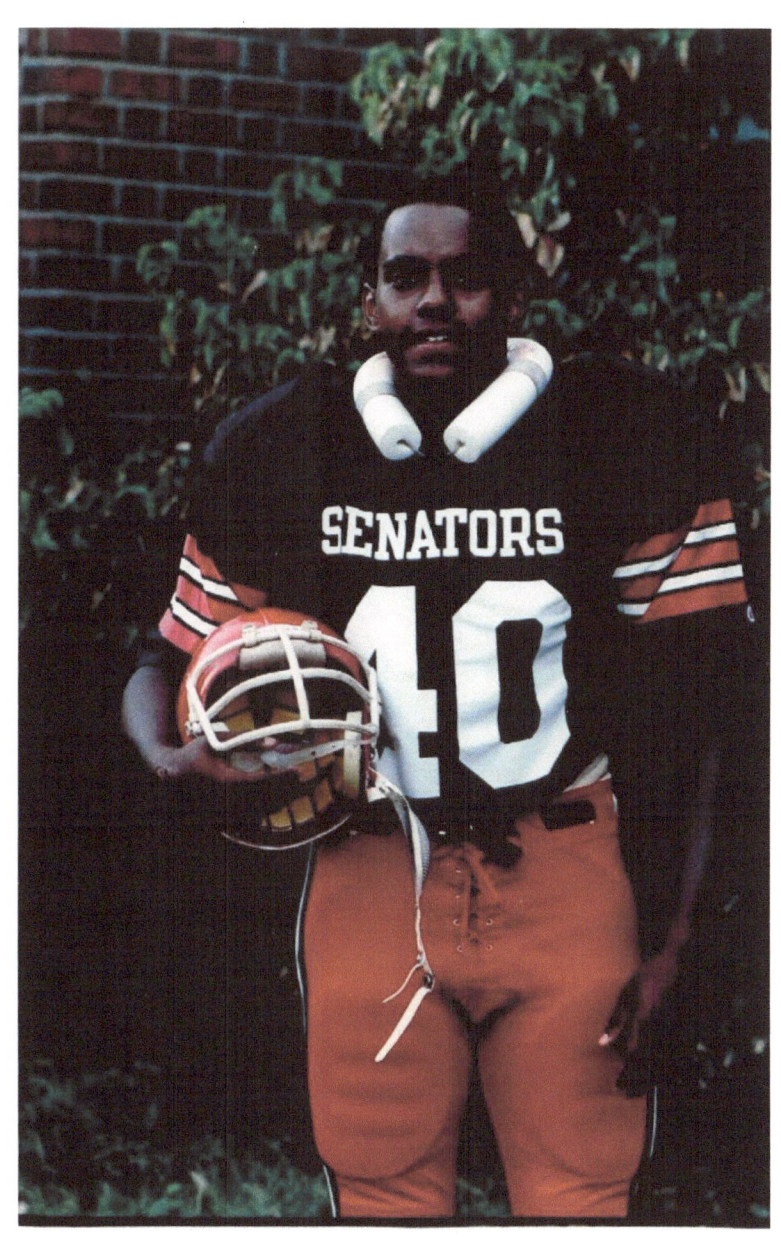

(Striper No More...High School Senior)

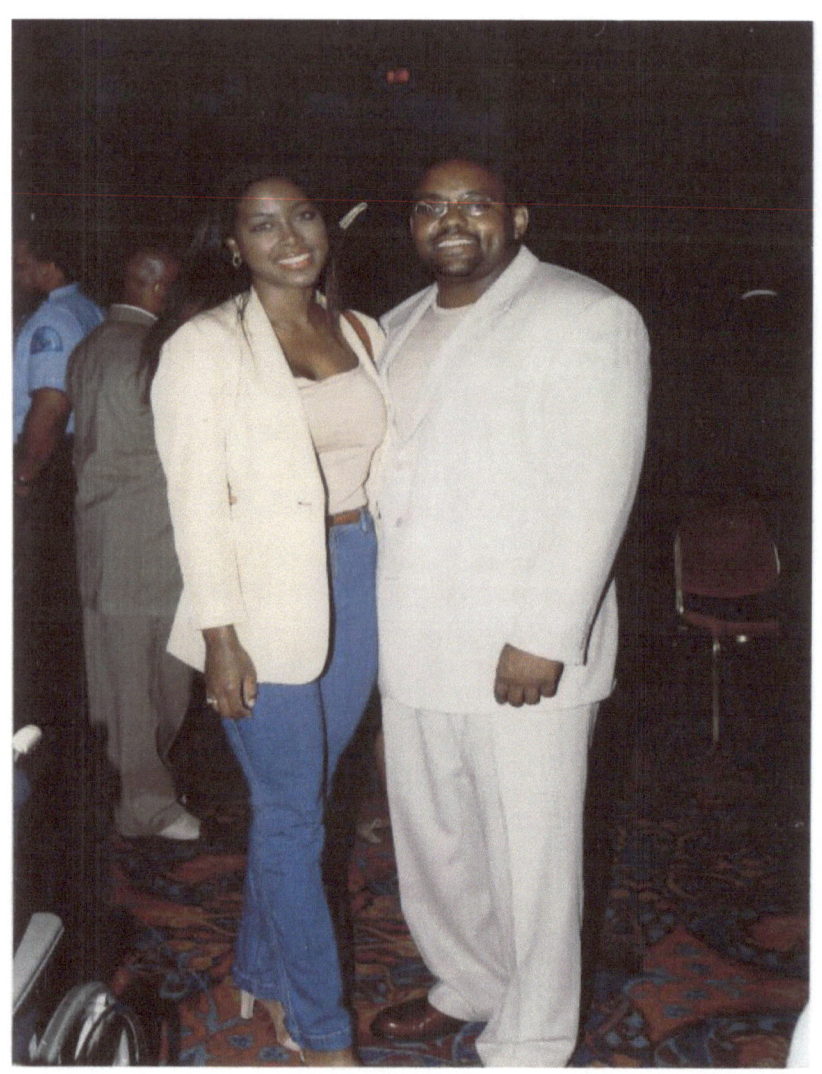

Throwback Picture: Me and Kenya Moore in the 90's

Long before she was crazy on the reality show "The Real Housewives of Atlanta" I met a kinder, gentler Miss USA 1993, Kenya Moore.

The Diet See Saw

After my striper years I became the guy who enjoyed working out and that routine became an important part of my life. I played football and ran track in high school and during my community college years I worked at the YMCA and was on the track team. This extended to my early years in the radio business too. In Huntsville, Alabama, I worked in health clubs not because I needed the money but because I enjoyed the environment of the gym.   Now keep in mind that I was maintaining what I thought was my ideal fitness level at this time but I would soon have a rude awakening.   One day I when I was running in Huntsville I caught a glimpse of myself in a window and I noticed the few extra pounds I was carrying.   I also remember doing hanging crunches and looking in the mirror and instead of seeing my tight fat free stomach I saw a layer of fat covering my midsection, it was a sign of things to come.   When I started working I started having less time for working out and staying in shape.   Again, at this point I was still in relatively good shape but I was losing my fitness level I had established in college.   I started endorsing different diets on the radio (I believe Nutri-system was the first one I did back in the 90's).   They would give you these dehydrated meals like a hamburger that you would put in a hot bowl of water and then eat.   The diets worked but I believe what happened over time was I would lose 20 to 40 pounds of muscle on these various diets and then gain back 20 to 40 pounds of fat.   Over time this changed my metabolism.   Over the years I endorsed most all the diet products that were out there including Nutri-system, Metabolife, Weight Watchers, LA Weight loss and The Adkins diet.   They all worked but I believe this gaining and losing weight contributed to my overall weight gain.   For the most part I stayed in good shape from High School to College with my fighting weight being around 200 pounds.   After college in my first job in Huntsville Alabama I was the Program Director, Morning Show host and the Production Director and along with the responsibility of the new job came a pager, remember them?, The stress of being a manager meant extra stress and that stress meant more weight.   After Huntsville I moved to Charleston SC and started doing Mornings.   Since I was no longer in management the stress was gone and again I had more time to work out.   I hit the gym hard again and the wonderful climate of South Carolina contributed to me getting back in great shape.   I really do believe the fact that I was at the beach at least three times a week contributed to me being more aware of my beach body and my overall health.   After Charleston I headed to St Louis where instead of hitting the beach three times a week, I was hitting the BBQ shack!   I had a great time but I also got comfortable and plenty of comfort food to boot.   Late nights at White Castle and Steak and Shake, The famous Saint Paul sandwich (which was and egg sandwich on white bread with mayo), Mother's fish, Sarah Lou's hamburgers, The Best Steak across from the Fox Theatre, Ted Drew's frozen custard, Church's Chicken, Bojangles, I could go on and on.   In St Louis I also endorsed various weight loss programs and lost and gained over the years with my weight sliding up and down between 220 and 270.   What I didn't know was that I would go on to gain at least sixty more pounds and would soon hear the devastating pre diabetes diagnosis.

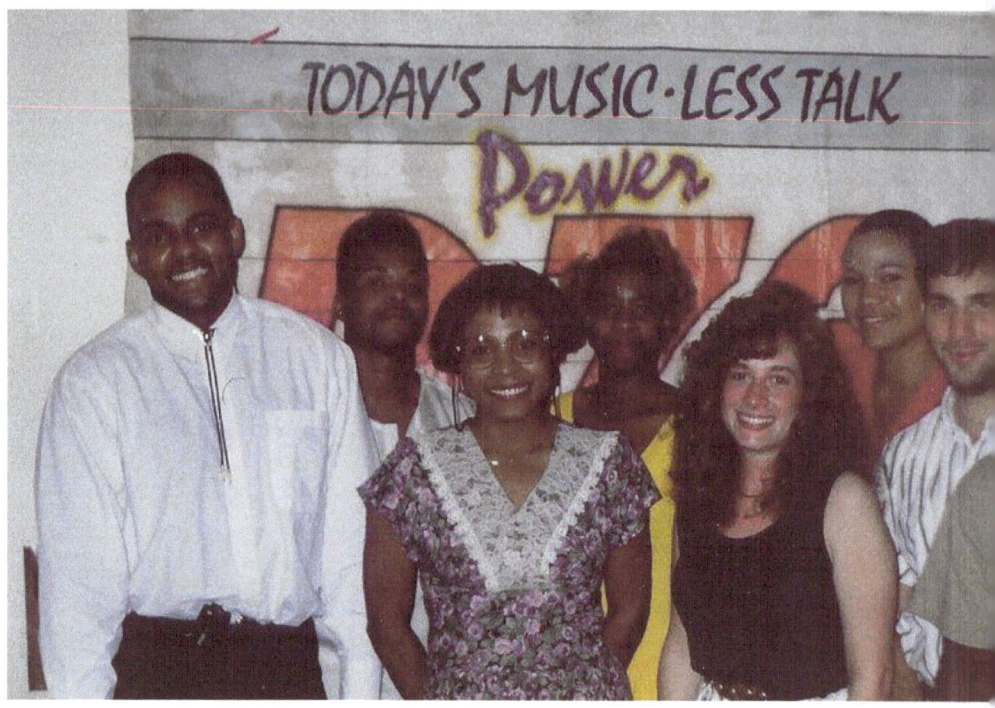

In Huntsville, Alabama at Power D-73 AM my first Morning radio job after college. I was in good shape physically but style- wise I may have been in trouble.

THE FINAL STRAW, THE MOMENT, THE BREAKING POINT

After the visit to the doctor, I decided then to change my life drastically. First I cut out the carbohydrates. I ate fruits and vegetables but cut out all of the bread, rice, pasta, potatoes, soda, and juice. All the carbs had to go because I was a bit paranoid and did not want to set myself up for diabetes. I also started exercising at least thirty minutes a day again understanding that this was a way to defend against diabetes. Two weeks after I visited the doctor on the return visit I was about fourteen pounds lighter but she said my blood pressure still was not where she wanted it to be. What she did not know is I stopped taking the blood pressure medicine because I felt like it was harming my body. I didn't know how, but I felt like blood pressure drugs along with cholesterol drugs were not good for my system. I did not have any research but it was just my feeling and I had a home BP monitors to make sure I was not out of control. My friend Troy Johnson turned me on to the movie "Sick, Fat and nearly dead" the story of a guy who did the 60 day juice cleanse and regained his health. He also followed the journey of a truck driver who tipped the scale at over four hundred pounds and lost well over one hundred pounds in sixty days of juicing. A friend had interviewed Carl Douglin from www.rawrawlife.com and was thinking about juicing. At that point I wasn't against it but I wasn't sure. I reached out to one of my closest friends who happen to be a kick ass nutritionist and trainer. He said I should do a cleanse first and he gave me the ingredients to get started.

THE PICTURE

I CALLED THIS PICTURE THE F.G.W.U.C.

The Fat Guy Wake up Call. When I saw this picture I knew something had to change. Here was my fly, sexy wife looking all young and vibrant and I was looking like somebody's Daddy, which I was but I was not ready to look like I was auditioning for the role of the "good reverend" quite yet. I still wanted to keep my youthful swag...

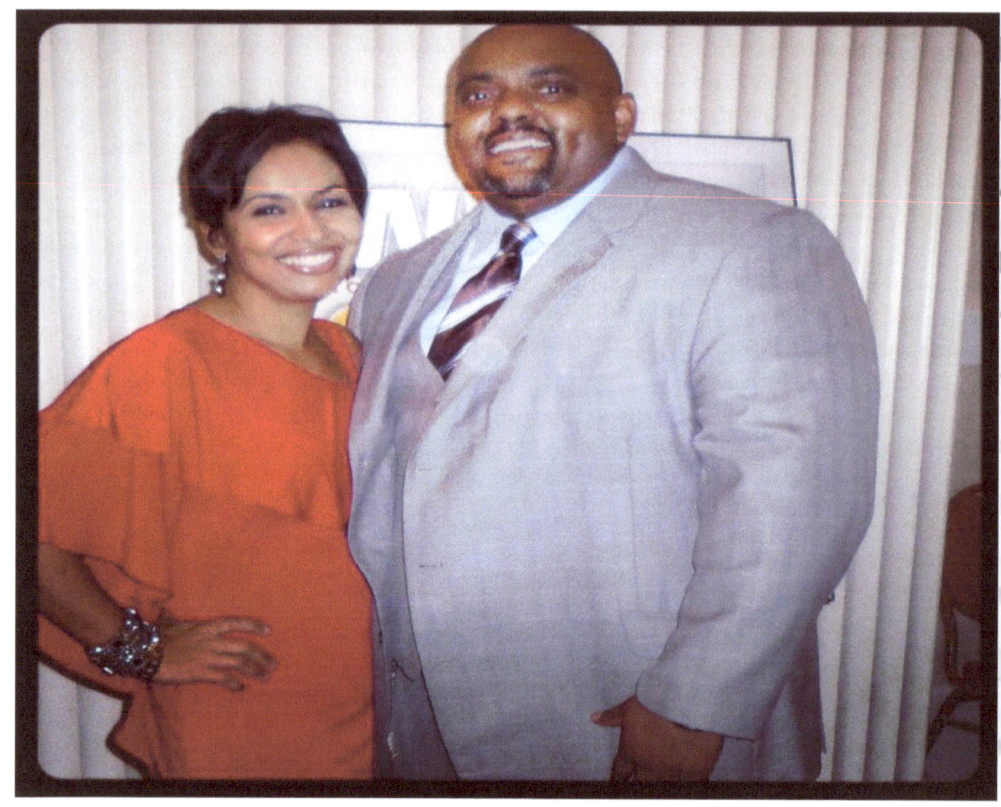

Fat.Guy.Wake.Up.Call!

THE PRE CLEANSE

The ingredients for the cleanse were lemons, distilled water, apple cider vinegar, black strap molasses, and cayenne pepper. There are a lot of cleanses out their but this one is great because it contains minerals and vitamins, it helps to make your system more alkaline vs. acidic. It does not taste bad. I was going to do seven day cleanse just to get a feel for it and it went surprisingly well. So well in fact that I decided to extend the cleanse to ten days. By the ninth day I had lost fourteen pounds and I received a call from my new employer that required me to leave for Qatar the next day. The last minute trip was the only reason I wrapped the cleanse earlier than I had hoped. I was on the plane the next day and my goal for the week was to break the fast correctly so I would not get ill especially on the plane for the eighteen hour flight. On that tenth day I did not eat anything but by dinner time I did start eating real

16

food starting with a salad. Each day I added more vegetables and then more fruits and then raw foods only and by Thursday I added eggs to my mix. By the weekend I was eating foods again without any problems. After doing the cleanse I had no doubt that I could do the juice cleanse. It would be better because of the variety of tastes that fruits and vegetables offer and I would go on my juicing journey with a group of colleagues. We agreed to start in July which was also the start of my family vacation. There's nothing like drinking your meals while driving to Florida to begin a Disney vacation! I knew this would prove to be an interesting experience. So many hurdles were in front of me. Would I fall to temptation? Could I make time to Juice while on the road? Could I resist the turkey Leg? These questions would all be answered at Disney World.

CARLA'S TOOL KIT ON HOW TO GET READY FOR AND START A FAST

I was so blessed to meet Carla Douglin. Carla was there for us all the way from showing us how to embark on our pre-fast to sharing her amazing book *101 Juice Fast Recipes* (which became my juice bible). Here is some of the information she provided to us to get started:

HOW TO PREPARE FOR A JUICE FAST

As mentioned in the Ten Tips section of *101 Juice Fast Recipes*, it is so important to ease your way into a juice fast. My suggestion: take one full week before your fast to make the switch. During this week, do NOT eat out. Plan to make your own food each and every day.

Beginning on Sunday, cut out processed foods from your diet and increase your water intake by 2 quarts/liters a day.

On Wednesday, begin eliminating all diary items and meat (milk, butter, cheese) from your diet.

On Friday, cut out the cooked food and begin eating the foods that you will be juicing during your fast-lots and lots of fresh fruits and veggies! Also, increase your water intake another quart/liter.

By Sunday, you are ready to begin your fast! Feel free to adjust those times and days as you see fit (you can even extend the timeframe to two weeks instead of one) but understand that this sample transition plan will help make your fast much easier.

Note: You may feel the need to have "One last meal" of junky foods, before beginning your juice fast or transition. This is definitely not a good idea, because your body doesn't understand the concept of time, and will still be trying to process and get rid of the junky "food" when you're transitioning. In fact, depending on how healthy your digestion is (and how often you empty your bowels), it can take many days to move out!

Also, as soon as you wake, begin each day with a glass of warm water with the juice of half a lemon in it. This helps prep the body and assists in cleansing your liver. Tip: If you keep your lemons at room temperature, and then roll it between your hand and a flat surface before squeezing, you will get much more juice from the lemon, and it will be easier to squeeze.

CHECK LIST TO GET STARTED

1. **Juicer**: I suggest a centrifugal juicer to get started (like a Breville). I love masticating juicers, but they take a lot of time to prep your juice, and we need to ensure you guys can juice, prep and go!

2. **Mason Jars**: I recommend the following jars, as they are 32 ounces and have a wide mouth (easier for pouring and cleaning) - http://amzn.to/J5s8GQ

3. **Thermos**: These Kleen Canteens are great to use for juice on the go. They are larger than mason jars (40 or 64 ounces to allow a greater amount of juice), BPA-free and, because they are stainless steel, keep juice fresh in the fridge longer. http://amzn.to/K1eLvp

4. **10 Tips Videos**: Take a look through the videos. Most importantly, check out the video for transitioning into a fast. This is the plan I'm going to take you two through the week before we get started. http://rawrawlife.com/newbies/juicenewbie/

HOW TO START A FAST

THE POWER OF FOCUS

The decision to fast for 60 days is just like the world of business in that every day there is a new opportunity to succeed or fail. Your intention is to have success but if you let your mind stray or are undisciplined you will fail. Every day has to be taken one day at a time and your success is an accumulation of your daily success. You are driven by your long term goals but if you don't accomplish your daily goals the long term will not happen. Visualization and dreaming are a huge part of your success. If you can't see yourself in 60 days, you are not visualizing success. Faith is belief in something not seen, or seen by your mind's eye only. How do I feel? I feel good. Not powerful, not weak but, less powerful. I'm visualizing my body burning fat.

THE START OF THE FAST

http://youtu.be/LEDoMh3BbLw

(Video featuring me and Troy and Carla starting the fast)

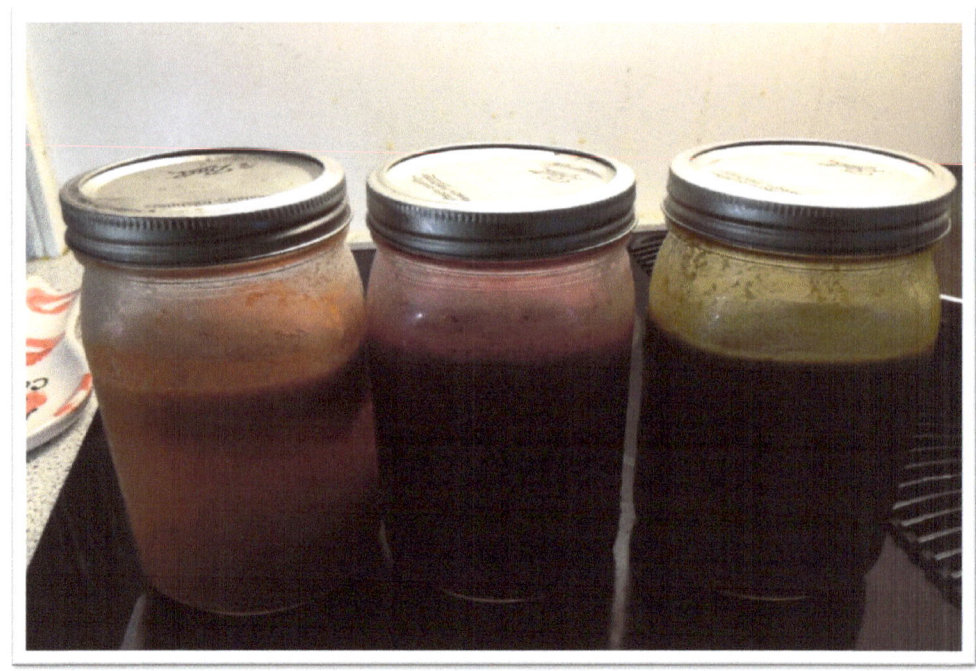

(Breakfast, Lunch Dinner)

The First 30 Days

The first 30 days of the Juice fast went without a hitch. The first few days are the hardest as your body adjusts to not eating and you really start to realize how much time you spend thinking about, preparing, and even planning transportation around eating. Now that you juice in the morning or the previous evening you have your food for the day and don't need to spend any more time on it. I would juice three thirty two ounce mason jars for each day and I would be set. I would pack them up in a cooler with ice and be on my way to work. Sometimes I would take a sixty four ounce thermos and take a mason jar and put it in the refrigerator at work. I took my juicer with me on vacation and even juiced in hotel rooms on many occasions. I was sticking to the plan by any means necessary.

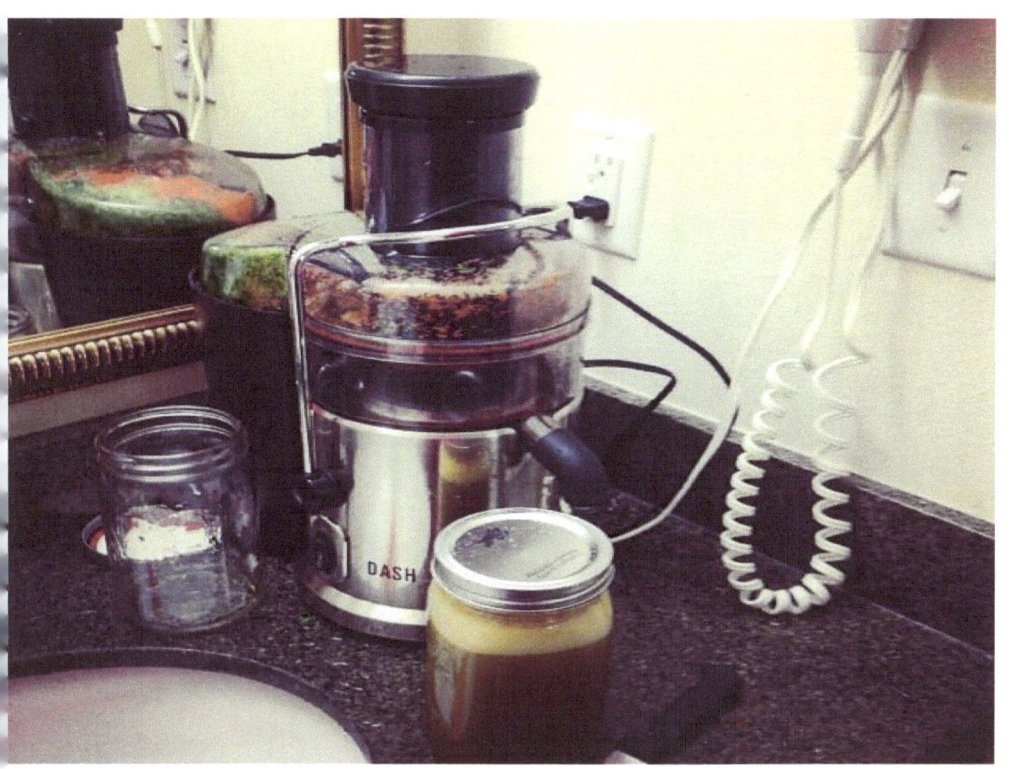

Have Juice will travel...my juicer on vacation

HALF WAY THERE!

http://youtu.be/kT-WMYUL41E

(The above link will take you a video of me and the group at the 30 day mark. Juice Fasting: The #Juice60 Halfway Mark!)

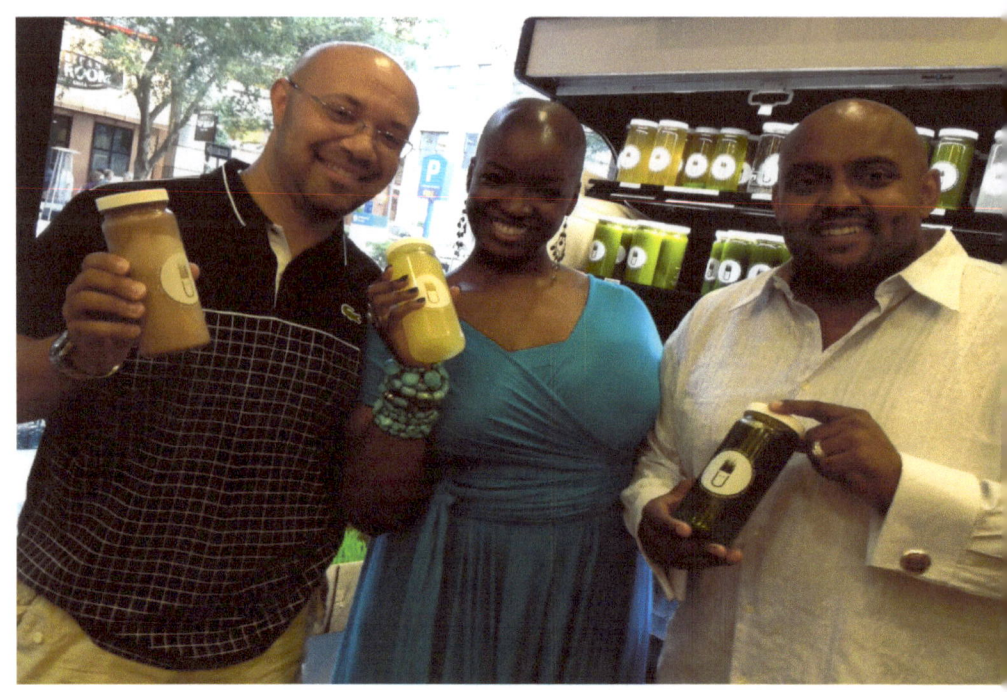

(From left to right: Troy Johnson, Carla Douglin, Marc Clarke)

We had a 30 juice fast happy hour and everyone kept asking how I felt. I definitely feel great about myself. One of the questions Carla and many others had was "Don't you feel so much better now that you've lost this weight?" and initially my answer was "Well not really, I always felt good." They would say "Don't you have so much more energy?" and I would say "I've always had a lot of energy." I think this speaks to a little bit of denial I had when I was not my fit self. When the guy that I used to be or desired to be wasn't the guy I was looking at in the mirror. I told myself that everything was good, when it really was not. After the 30 day party, we had another party at Puree juice bar in Bethesda. We had that conversation on Saturday night's radio program with Carla and Amy and when I walked on Sunday I had to admit to myself that I did feel much better. I felt lighter, a little more energized, a little bit more pep in my step. The truth is that after this weight loss, I did, in fact, feel better. Furthermore, the feeling better is feeling better about me. I think when you start gaining weight one of the tale tell signs is when you are on vacation and the wife wants to take pictures and you start finding yourself not wanting to be in any pictures because none of them are acceptable to you , you don't like the way you look. Subconsciously it starts to affect you. I could tell I was getting my swagger back when I would walk out of the shower and in front of my wife without making sure I was covered up in the robe tied tightly around my midsection. I was feeling better about myself and feeling better internally. When you're not where you think you should be, even if you don't admit it to yourself, it has an effect not only on you but on others close to you too. So after losing 37 pounds on the fast and a total of 60 pounds since I found out from the Doctor I was pre-diabetic I definitely was feeling better about me. I would use Phase two to expedite these great feelings and the weight loss and the fitness. In phase two I started to step up my fitness by walking every morning. Get up early (6:00am), weigh, get in a mile or two, and do a series of calisthenics each morning.

During the fast I would often awake feeling guilty because in my dreams I would have just devoured a whole rack of ribs and my lips and mouth would still be tingling with the taste of Smokey barbeque sauce, the pepper mixed with the Smokey, sweet taste of bbq sauce so I would also have the piece of white bread to take care of that. Or I remember the first time I had one of those dreams it was fried chicken. I woke up feeling satiated and you know how it is. It's hard to find good fried chicken in reality and in your dreams.

Day 40

I was moving along on the fast and happy with the progress of my health and especially the weight loss. I did not want to promote this as a way to lose weight. I instead wanted to use the juice fast as a way to get control of my diet and in that process lose weight as a side effect of controlling my food intake. Wow, seeing these words makes it sound like a bunch of crap but I was concerned that everybody would want to fast just to lose weight and not really focus on the power of raw fruits and vegetables and the benefits. At the end of the day people really just want to know how to lose weight. So as I approached day forty of the juice fast I had the thought that at the end of sixty days I will be around 248 pounds. A significant loss as my original pre fast weight was 330 but then I asked the question, was that enough. I wanted to lose at least 100 pounds and that would put me at around 230. I knew that when I stopped the juice fast I would not be taking this type of journey again anytime soon so I had the thought that maybe I should go 100 days. That way when I finished I would be more around the 220's. Well, it's funny how life works, I was scheduled to do a sleep study because a new client, Rest Assured, needed a radio personality to endorse the product and since I was big they assumed that I would fit the profile. Turns out they were absolutely right. The sleep study concluded that I had mild sleep apnea. One of the ways to get rid of it was to lose weight, in my case about 25 to 30 pounds. So again I thought about extending the juice fast to 100 days. I built such a great relationship with the staff at Rest Assured and learned so much about the dangers of sleep apnea and how it could be treated and save lives that I wanted not only to talk about it on the radio but to get the message out any way that I could. I eventually became an advocate for sleep apnea awareness.

,

ALMOST THERE

As I went deep into day forty and beyond, I again had thoughts about doing 100 days. I knew that many people who were inspired by the film "Sick, Fat, and Tired" were doing the 60 day fast and I thought hey why not go for 100 days? I would lose more weight and when I started eating again I would not be as concerned when I started the natural process of gaining weight because I was eating whole food. I loved losing the weight but after working out at the gym and looking in the mirror I realized that the weight loss process for me was going to be three phases; losing the fat and the weight, building back the core muscles with cardio and resistant exercise, and maintaining the new body. I realized that losing the weight in many ways could be the easiest part of the equation. Reshaping the body after losing around 100 pounds is quite a challenge but the discipline I developed through fasting would help me stay focused. I decided to do just 60 days.

Home Stretch

Around day fifty I started to look forward to chewing food again and I had the strangest craving. When I went to Whole Foods to get my fruits and veggies I would always be drawn to the sample of guacamole with chips and I could not wait until I could finally get my guac on. The funny thing was I just wanted to eat some guacamole out of the container with no chips. I probably was craving that good natural fat. And don't you know the first thing I had when I broke the fast was guacamole? I was so proud of myself at this point in the fast. I learned the power of focus and fortitude. I also learned that people are really inspired when they see someone then know personally make a positive change in their life especially something like weight loss. People did not say it but they were worried about my weight and seeing me do this made them happy for me and my family. The reaction on Facebook when I posted pictures was startling with hundreds of comments and thousands of likes. I could not wait to wrap up the fast but I also knew I had to write about this amazing experience.

Power of words

Going on the fast with a group really helped me stay focused. I had agreed to do it and wanted to keep my word. In Wayne W. Dyer's book "Manifest Your Destiny" he addresses the power of words. He says:

"Make your word law! If you say it, live up to it lovingly. This gives you a sense of inner balance this is missing in those who live with self-repudiation and guilt. The more you practice 'My word is law. I must keep it,' the more balanced your life becomes.

The universe runs on balance, and the energy that keeps it in balance is love. By declaring yourself as a person who keeps his word, you align yourself with the loving essence of the world."

In those moments that I wanted to quit the fast I was motivated by my agreement with the others that we would go the distance, together.

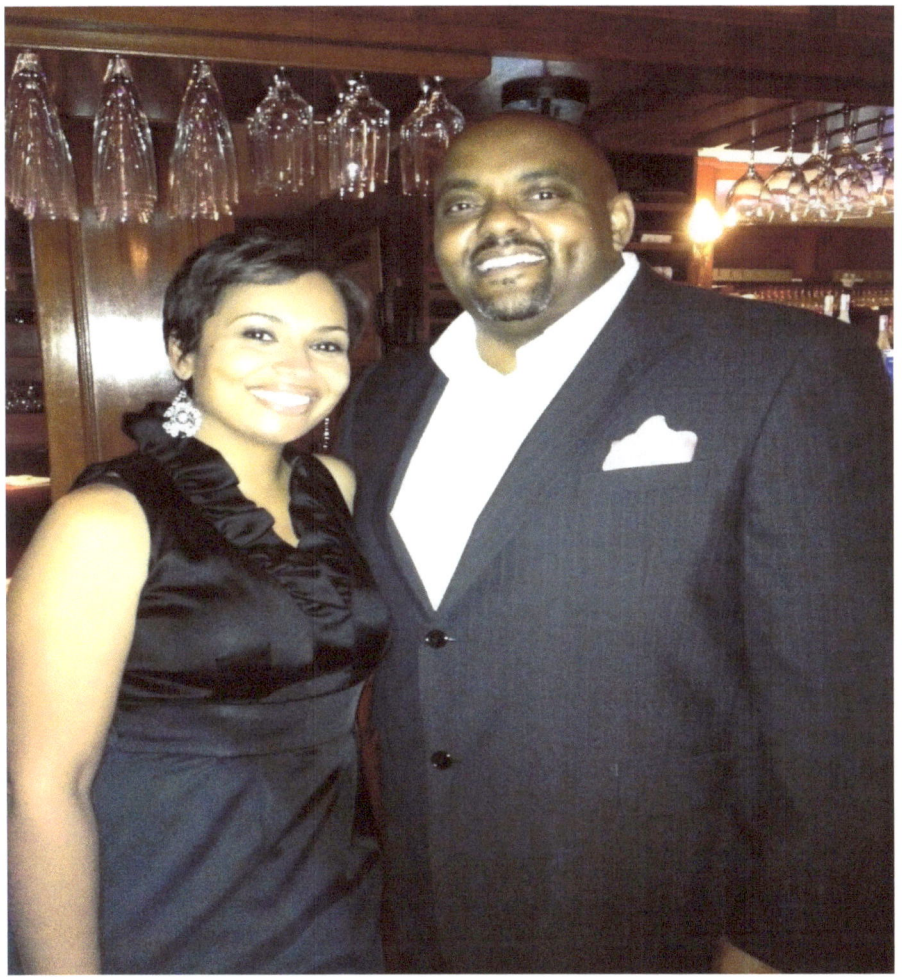

Me and Allison around Day 40

Allison and I at Jason Murphy's Holding the line Foundation fundraiser in Baltimore, MD. I had on one of my new suits down one size and feeling good.

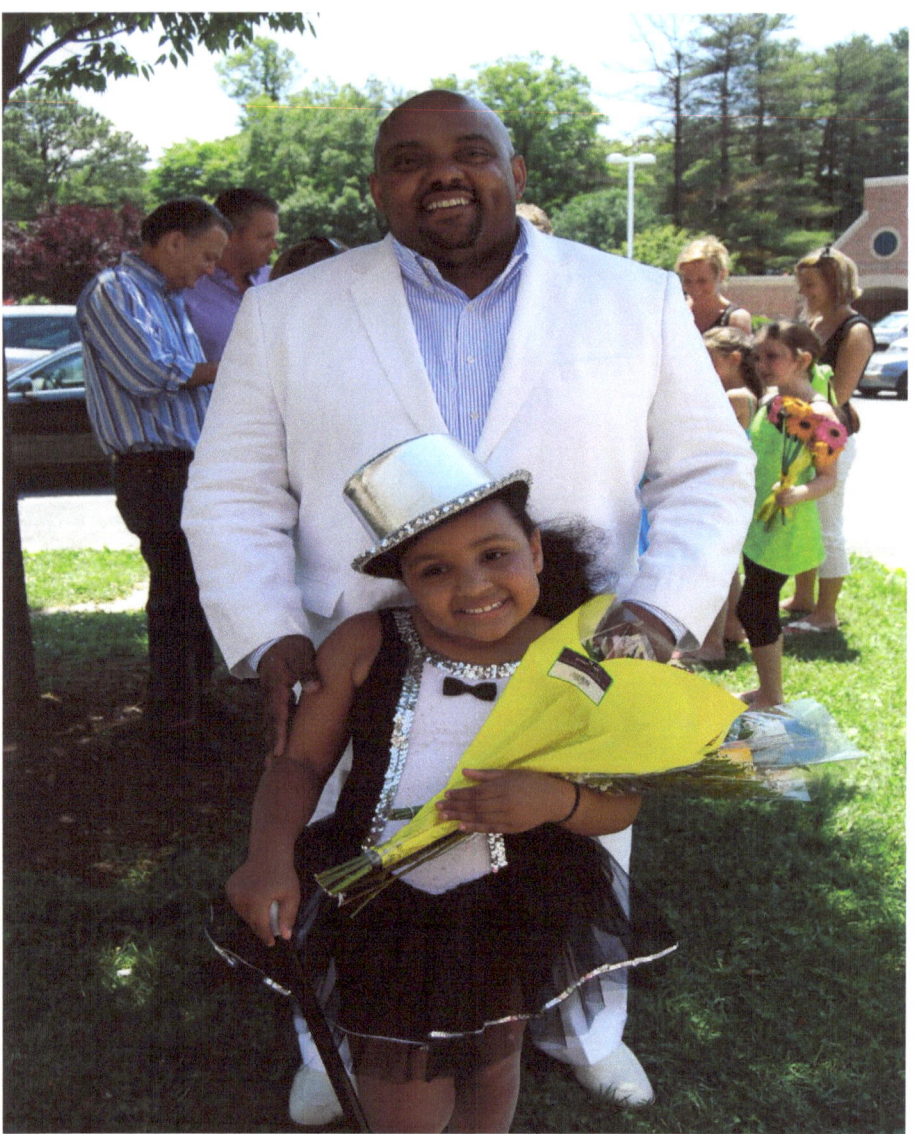

I think the white suit does make me look bigger

My youngest daughter Spencer and me after her dance recital. I had on my new white suite and thought I was looking good.

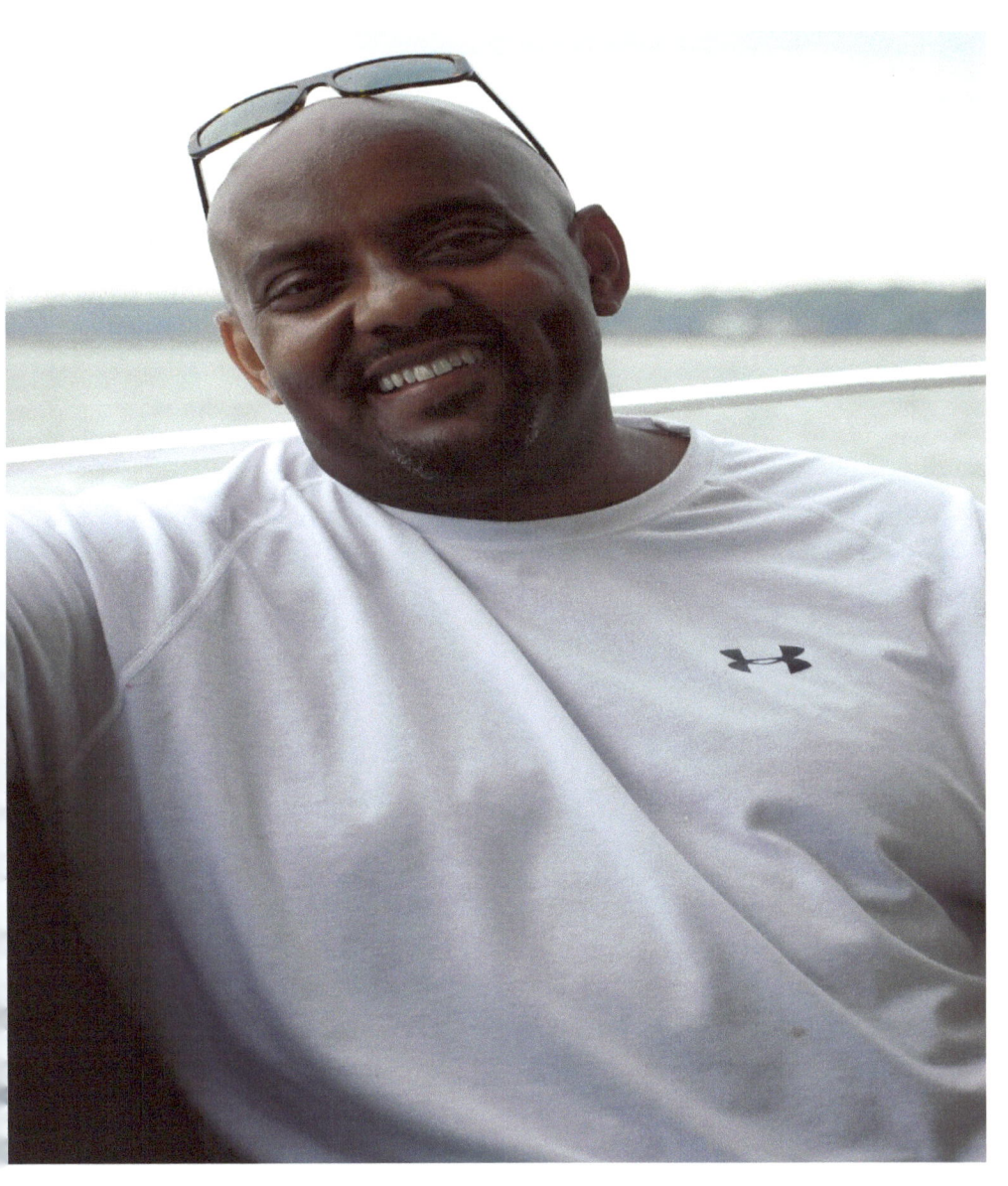

Getting my swagger back!

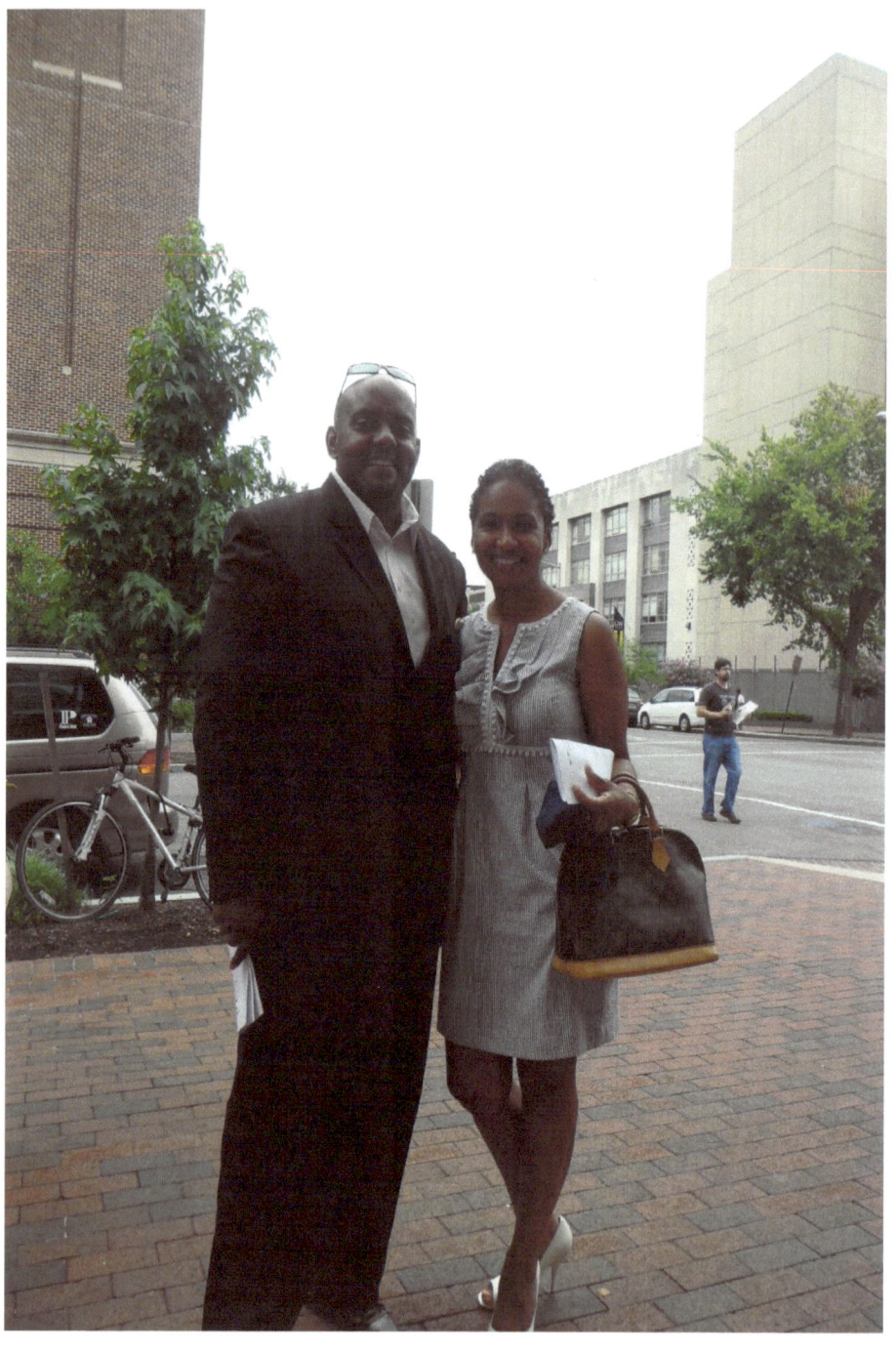

We've come a long way baby!! My best friend and most vigilant supporter, Allison

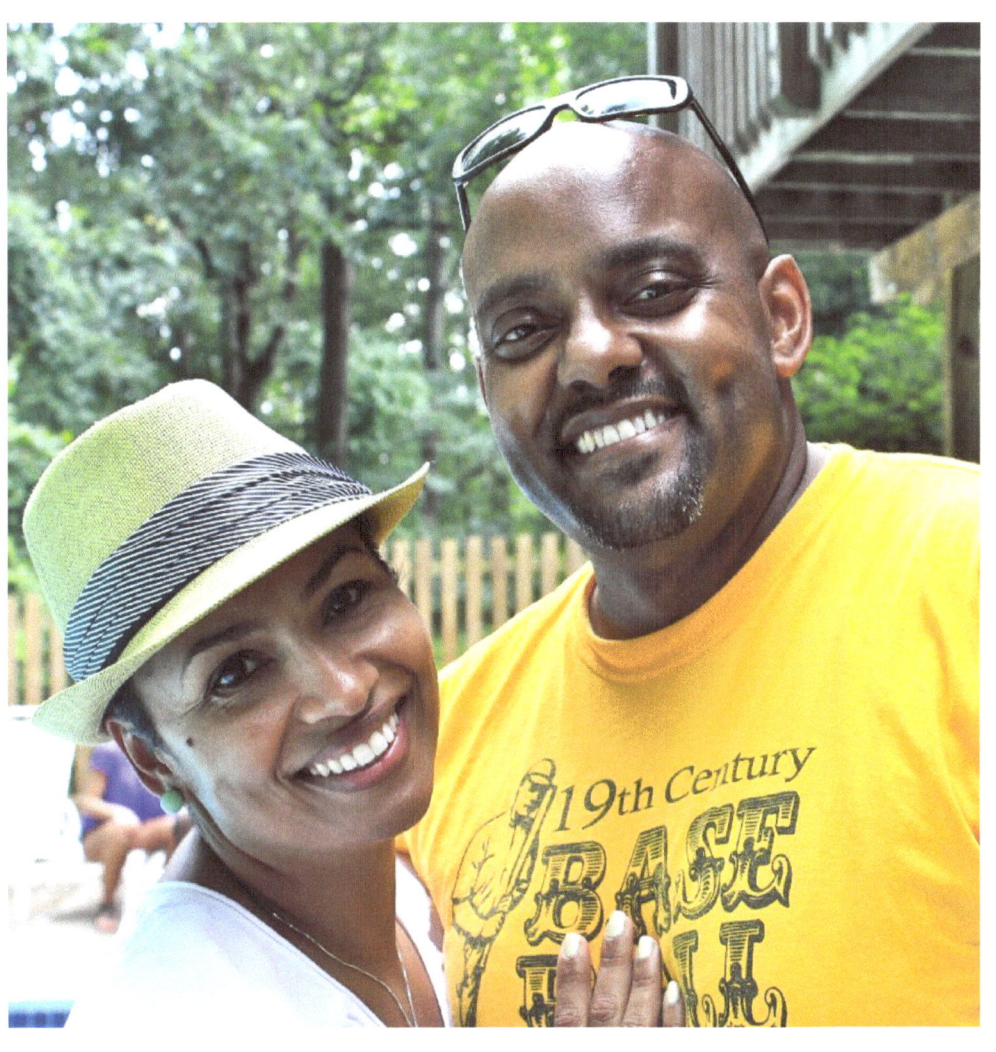

Living Again!

The 60 day fast put me back in touch with my inner warrior. It was always there but I had lost my way. I was always competitive in life and had a no quit mentality but I got lulled into slowly letting go of managing myself and demanding excellence in myself. I picked up bad habits including, Procrastination, lack of focus, settling, lack of drive, not paying attention to detail, lack of order and complacency. I had to be reminded of who I was and how I achieved the goals that make me successful. I am now revitalized and ready to face the second half of life. It starts with your health. If you don't have your health, nothing else matters. If you manage what you eat you probably are more inclined to manage your spiritual life, business, family, job, everything. The saying "you are what you eat" is more than a cliché it really is a life changer. As I was eating all healthy organic fruits and vegetables I felt a certain power and strength knowing that I was not putting anything bad in my body. I have a certain confidence and I am healthy and in control. I can't imagine giving this feeling up to go back to bad food. I have more energy for playing with the kids, creating wealth for my family, spirituality, giving back to the community, loving my wife, building and taking care of my friendships, walking the dogs, everything. Passion is back in my life. No meds.

TALE OF THE TAPE

	BEFORE	AFTER
WEIGHT:	328	250
BLOOD PRESSURE:	145/90	115/65
NECK:	21	17.5
CHEST:	57	51
HIPS:	56	45
STOMACH:	56	46

WHAT I'VE LEARNED

At the end of the 60 days I weighed 250 pounds and had a new outlook on life. I was twenty pounds from my 100 pound weight loss goal but had no doubt that I would get there. Phase two was to get rid of the jangly fat and loose skin around my midsection and to do this I was going to start training like I did years ago when I was young and hungry. I was excited about this challenge. Here are a few things I learned about myself and about life during this juice fast:

Juicing was the most effective and efficient form of weight control that I have tried.

I've learned to appreciate the nutritional power of fruits and vegetables

I feel more at peace with the universe and understand the importance of preserving healthy organic farming and fruits and vegetable. I am also more aware of all of the cancer causing agents in our foods and environment.

I try to prepare the most nutritionally dense food for myself and my family

I love shopping for new clothes in stores where I could not before and I use this to motivate me to stay focused

I think people are surprised at my style of dress. For so many years I could not reflect who I always wanted to be because the clothes were either too expensive or did not come in my size

HOW TO BREAK YOUR FAST

Once again I turned to Carla Douglin for advice on how to break the fast in a healthy manner she has an amazing book called "How to Break a Juice Fast" by Carla Douglin with Awanda Baker that I recommend for a healthy transition out of the juice fast. I started with juices, smoothies and broths before moving onto soft fruits and salads. As a rule, it should take one third the amount of time you fasted to transition, which for a sixty day fast is about three weeks. You want to take your time and not hurt your system by eating too soon. Juicing no doubt added twenty to thirty years onto my life. Good luck and happy juicing!

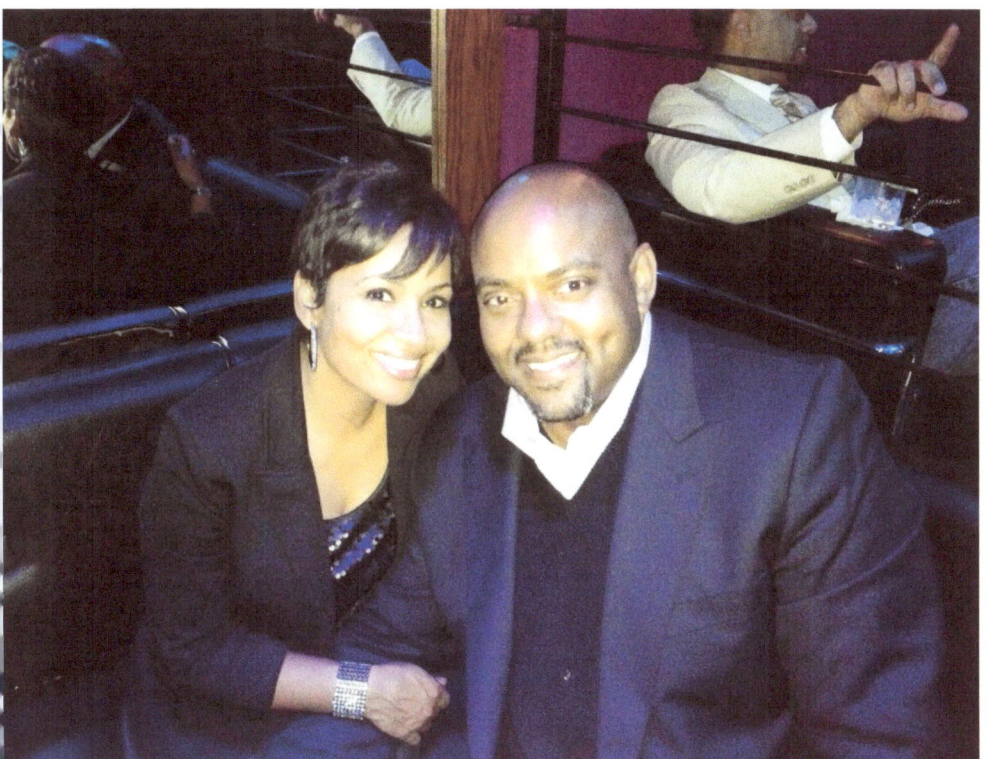

Maintaining Three months after the fast

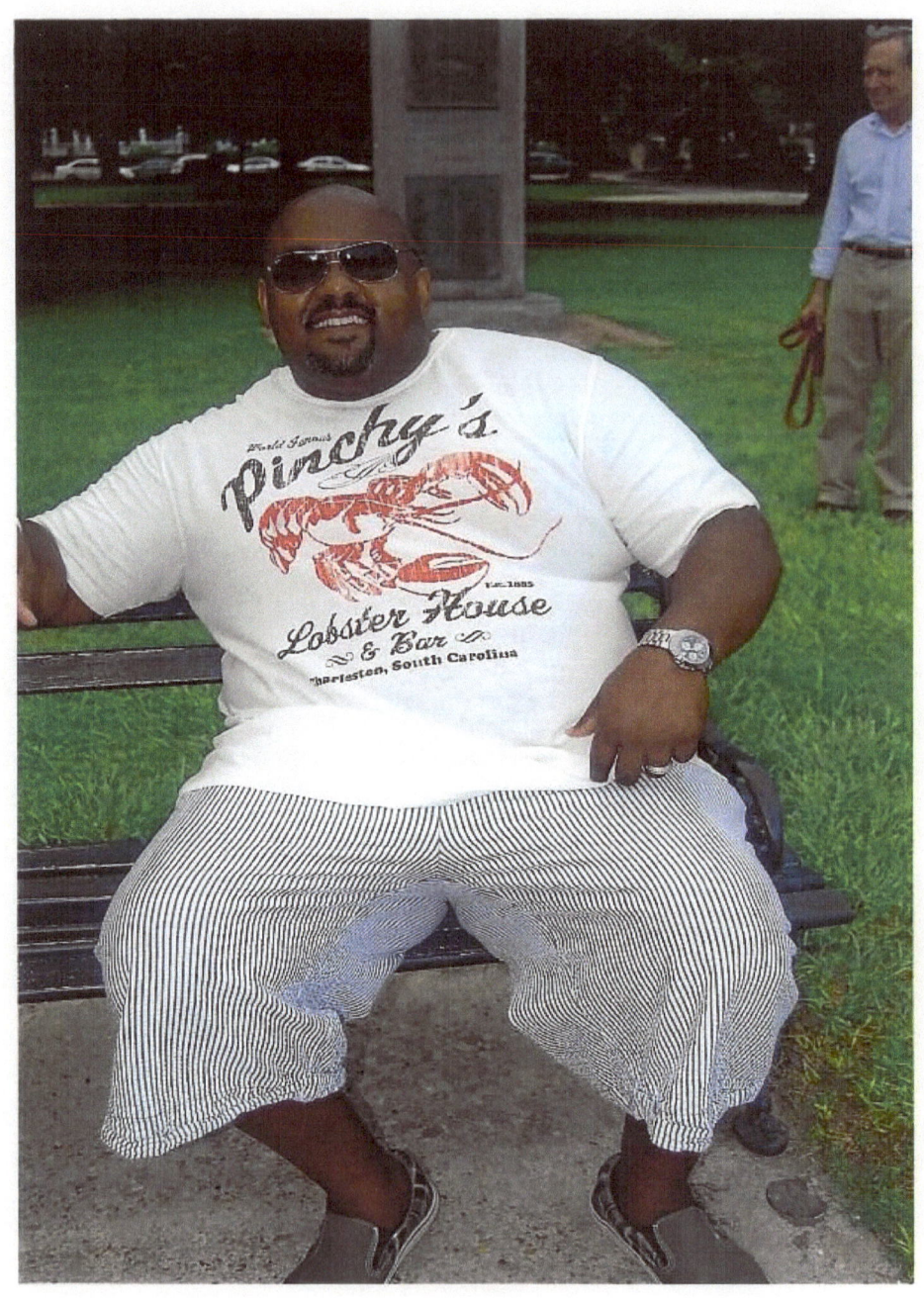

Before

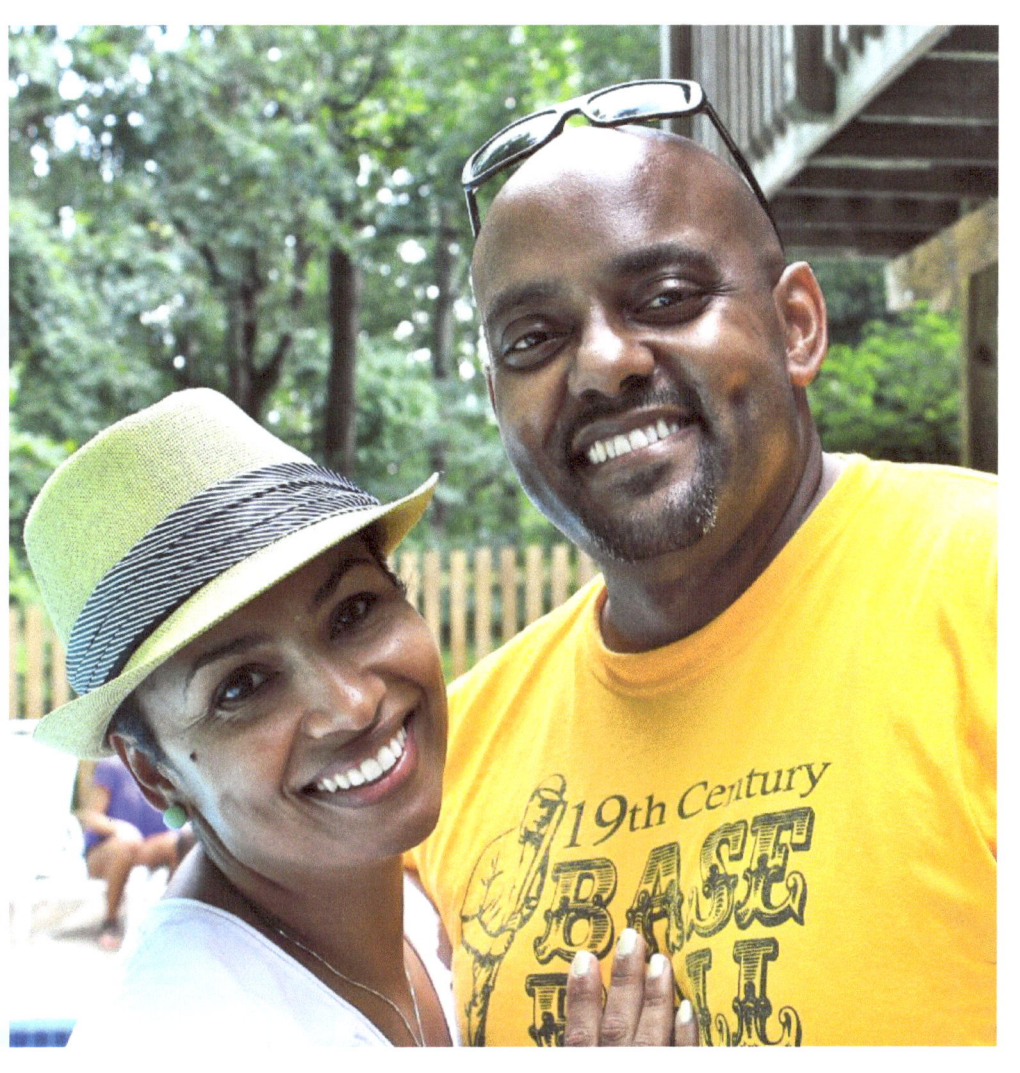

After

THE END